Cancer Prevention We

Malian Jasmine Lahey ©2023

Cancer prevention and wellness are not a substitute for advice from a doctor.

All information in this booklet should be vetted by your doctor, especially if you are already undergoing cancer treatment.

If you are taking SSRI medication (selective serotonin reuptake inhibitors) such as Prozac, Celexa, Zoloft, Lexapro, Paxil or others, you cannot take ginseng or herbal formulas containing ginseng. These drugs also have interactions with kava kava, MDMA, magic mushrooms and so on. Please keep yourself informed by asking your doctor about drug interactions.

TABLE OF CONTENTS

Order of operations and essential principles

This guide is structured so that first things come first. The order of the chapters is the order in which it's a good idea to proceed with cancer prevention.

That said, if you begin reducing inflammation, you can move on to the next step once you notice that the measures you took to reduce inflammation are taking effect, which can happen fairly quickly. You can then return to this step as needed.

Reducing and eliminating naturally comes before building and adding. Eliminating toxins needs to begin before adding herbs that interact with the endocrine system. Still, these are just rules of thumb. Listen to your own sense of what is going on with you and consult with your doctor. Eliminating toxins can be tricky if your cancer is metastatic. Avoid physically flushing the body with vigorous exercise or purgatives like Kambo frog poison or a liver or kidney flush and stick with gentle substances that chelate and render the toxins harmless, like turkey tail mushroom.

The general principles of restoring the balance of health in the body:

1. Reducing Inflammation and Antioxidants
2. Eliminate toxins from the body by flushing out with water based and oil based substances
3. Endocrine regulators
4. Build your immune system

Reduce inflammation
Reducing inflammation is partially avoiding things that cause inflammation. These can have emotional, energetic, environmental or

dietary causes that are mainly habitual, meaning we tend to tune out the wear and tear this puts on the bodymind.

Emotional causes can be:
- Getting angry, getting sad, qorking too much, forcing ourselves to be upbeat and high energy when we really need to rest. Dealing with an annoying or tiring situation we don't think we can change
- Something from the past that upsets us which we can't get closure from the other person because they have died, moved away, lost touch, etc.

Energetic causes can be:
- A lack of flow of energy in the body such as not saying what we think, not having sexual self expression, not moving the body and

getting exercise, not eliminating waste matter like menstrual blood, urine, feces, mucus, etc from the body.

- Giving our energy away habitually
- Hoarding our energy habitually

Environmental causes can be:

- Living near a trash incinerator or waste facility
- Agricultural or household chemicals
- Working with lead or petrol
- Bacterial or viral infection

Dietary causes can be:

- Excess consumption of alcohol
- Habitual consumption of meat that accumulates toxins such as agricultural chemicals or fish which eat other fish (such as

tuna)

- Habitual consumption of recreational substances especially those that are chemically processed

Reducing inflammation starts with eliminating these factors from one's experience and daily existence. Sometimes that takes a herculean effort, cost, and inconvenience. However the results are often miraculous. Laugh more, go to a counselor or therapist, talk to healers, sell your house and move away, etc. It's a quest, and you're a genius. You can do this!

Another side of reducing inflammation is increasing our intake to things that soothe our system. We have a network of "interstitial tissue" in our body, that white webby stuff that includes our lymph nodes and goes in between our organs and intestines. This stuff is loaded with white blood cells.

However when we have inflammation, the interstitial tissue starts to get damaged and that's a drag on our whole immune system. If we have chemicals in our bone marrow, where white blood cells are produced, that is a drag on our immune system. We want to support our immune system by getting enough rest and being gentle on our body both in terms of physical activity and what we put in.

Supplements and foods that reduce inflammation:

- *Turmeric*

- *Lion's mane, chaga, reishi and turkey tail mushrooms, powder, or extract*

- *Coconut oil*

- *Olive Oil*

- *Seaweeds (kelp, dulse, konbu, etc)*

- *Antioxidants*

Antioxidants are a fun topic in and of themselves. There are foods that are themselves antioxidants, and some probiotics that produce antioxidants. Oxidizings molecules like acrylamides or other "free radicals" carry around excess negatively charged electrons, meaning they tear DNA and cell organelles apart by donating electrons. Antioxidants soothe these scary molecules, usually by absorbing the extra electrons.

Think of your body not just as parts, but as if it were a bag of water and fat in which various substances dissolve. When you put something into your body, it changes the electrical properties of the contents of the body through chemical reactions.
You want your body to remain a nice steady pH of about 7.35 to 7.45. However, the pH is not uniform due to the clumps of fat (cell walls and organelles) and the parts of the body. We want all the nooks and crannies and surfaces of the body to have the right pH inside and out.

Antioxidants that are effective and commonly available include:

- Wheat grass juice!!!! This one is loaded.

- White tea and green tea. Become a tea nerd.

- Blueberry Powder

- Any strongly colored fruit usually has anthocyanin or lycopene in the coloration and these colors are antioxidants

- Leafy green vegetables such as spinach, kale, chard, broccoli

- Topical Magnesium oil

- Magnesium supplements

- Vitamin C (you can take as much as you want of this unless you have a kidney stone or kidney disease and it won't hurt your body or make you sick)

- Ginko Supplements

- Genistein Supplements

- Charcoal

- Cannabinol (releases oxytocin, the body's strongest antioxidant)

- Glutathione

Genistein is a special compound produced by rhizopus oligosporus, the fungal culture that makes tempeh. Tempeh and soy products fermented with r. Oligosporus contain genistein.

My favorite method of getting genistein involves buying tempeh starter, pouring a packet into a freshly opened 32 oz soy milk container, and letting it sit for a few weeks, then taking shots. The key to success is keeping everything sparkling clean so that your culture stays *just* r. oligosporus. No drinking out of the container, wash the lid with soap if you touch it to the countertop, etc.

Eliminate toxins from the body by flushing out with water based and oil based substances Eliminating toxins from the body is tricky. Much of your success will depend on how accurately you can identify what toxins you may have been exposed to.

As a side note, waste is eliminated as urine, feces, ear wax, mucus, and menstrual blood. Do not be shy about puking, diarrhea, or spitting.

It is gross, if you need to be private while eliminating please be everyone's guest. However you need to purge out the toxins somehow and it helps if you can joyously "let it go" without inhibition.

Say goodbye to all that!

Chelators:

Chelators have enzymes that wrap around the toxins and can safely be eliminated as waste. These are foundational.

Everyone can take chelators.

- Turkey tail, chaga, reishi and lion's mane mushrooms

- Charcoal powder

- Humic acid

- Fulvic acid

Water based flushes:

- White willow bark tea

- Nettle tea

- Echinacea tea

- Parsley tea

- Burdock tea

- Ajo Sacha tea

- Coffee enema or green coffee enema

The kidney cleanse from Hulda Clark's book "The Cure For All Diseases" is a water based flush.

Oil based flushes:

- Drink coconut oil or olive oil

- Drink milk combined with ghee

- Drink a few drops of eucalyptus oil dissolved in sesame oil. This will make you puke and you need a whole day to recover, but it goes all the way to the bone.

The liver cleanse from Hulda Clark's book "The Cure For All Diseases" is an oil based flush. Harsh flushes for toxins include the eucalyptus oil, Hulda Clark flushes and

Kambo frog poison. These can not be utilized if someone already has a cancer, especially one that is metastatic. They are for maintenance wellness purposes only.

Endocrine regulators

Herbs that are endocrine regulators rebalance and tone the hormones. Usually this stops harsh chemicals from messing with our system.

- Ashwaghanda
- Ginseng
- Turkey tail, chaga, reishi mushrooms

Endocrine regulators that deal with female hormones:

- Shatavari

- Dong Quai

Build Your Immune System

Our immune system is designed to destroy cancer. Every day our immune system finds and eliminates cancer from our bodies. If there is a cancer diagnosis, that means that either something is feeding the cancer or discouraging our immune system or both. Overcompensate by having a bangin' immune system.

The number one most helpful herb I have used is ginseng. Ginseng cannot be taken with certain antidepressants that are SSRIs and cannot be taken by people who have high blood pressure.

If these are not concerns for you, drinking ginseng tea four times a day is advised. Take ginseng tincture. You will feel the surge in your immune system.

Immune system herbs:

- Ginseng

- Echinacea

- Ginger

- Astragalus

- Burdock

- Echinacea

- Chili

- Cinnamon

You might be vegan or vegetarian and get grossed out by what I'm about to say, but eating bone broth or bone marrow could save your life. It is loaded with stem cells, which are what your body needs to produce white blood cells, killer T cells and leukocytes that destroy cancer and infection.

If you really want to stay vegetarian, make your own sourdough or ferments and eat the beneficial bacteria in there, which is almost as straightforward for your body to use as animal stem cells.

Acupuncture, tai chi, yoga, and other practices that calm down the sympathetic nervous system (fight or flight) and activate the parasympathetic (rest and digest), will support your immune system.

Conclusion

This is all information that I have tested on myself. You might have a different experience, but these methods are fairly tried and true. Trust your body to choose or reject any or all of these methods. Listen to yourself.

If you hate astragalus, don't worry. Make up for it with something else. If you just craaaave magnesium supplements or glutathione and drink it all day long, pay attention to that. Also pay attention when your body stops craving that and move on to something else.

Anyone can use these methods for better health. Keep educating yourself, ask a lot of questions, talk to your doctor, and most of all, LOVE YOURSELF.

Love releases oxytocin, the body's strongest antioxidant. Hugging, cuddling (but not orgasm) releases oxytocin. Having lots of caring people we don't touch but who show us we're important to them, releases oxytocin.

Our pets release oxytocin. Having fun and doing something that makes you smile releases oxytocin.

LOVE YOURSELF, LOVE YOURSELF LOVE YOURSELF.

Self care is not selfish. It is a sacred contract of honoring the divine spark within ourselves.

Blessings, love and light, Malian.

I've included pictures of my journey and experience in the following pages:

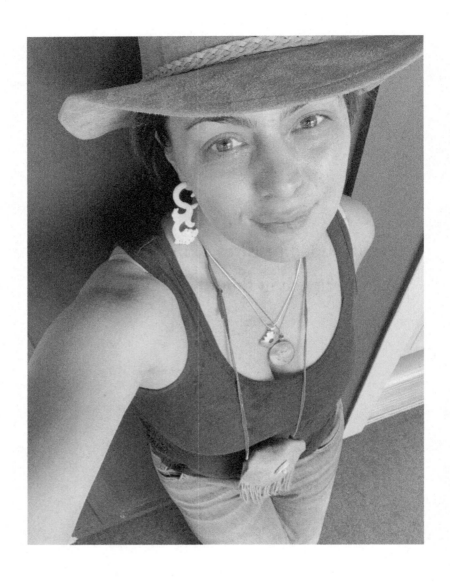

May 3, 2019 going to get my kidneys, liver, spleen and
blood checked in Reno, Nevada, U.S.A.

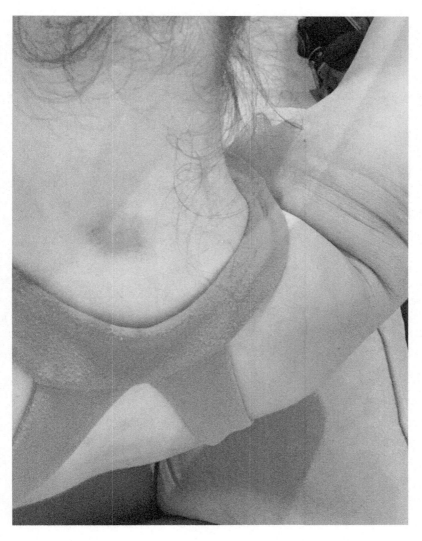

This was on June 27, 2019 poison being excreted through my skin.

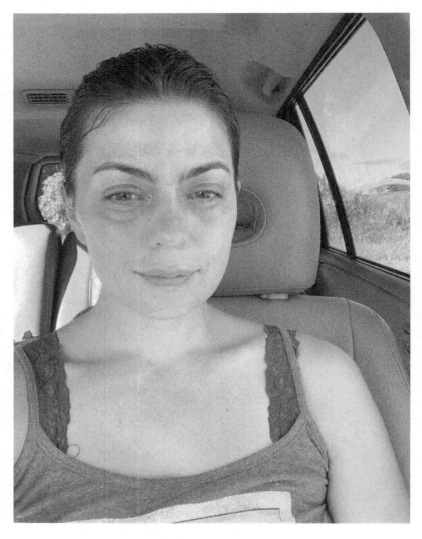

This was taken July 5, 2019, feeling sick and scared to die.

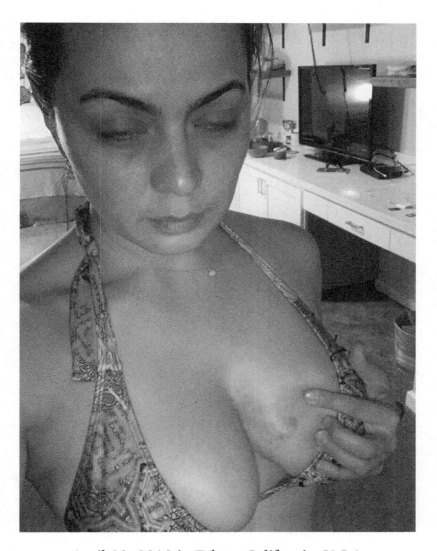

April 28, 2019 in Tahoe, California, U.S.A

Maestra Matilde at her retreat center in Peru.

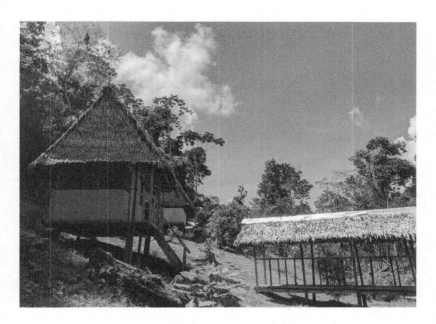

Maestra Matilde's retreat center in Peru.

The Cancer Prevention Kitchen

Recipes that Heal

Introduction To The Cancer Prevention Kitchen

If you have a serious commitment to lowering your risk of cancer, you're going to love these recipes! Our food is our medicine, as many of you well know and practice everyday.

These recipes are built around principles that support cancer prevention. Reducing meat, processed foods, heavy sauces, refined sugars, while increasing nutrient dense, antioxidant-rich foods will naturally support your body's innate ability to destroy cancer cells.

That said, it is still worth it to visit a professional nutritionist who can test your blood for allergies and food sensitivities. If nuts, milk, eggs, soy, or any other foods cause inflammation in your system, you need to know as soon as possible.

You would be surprised! I found out from a nutritionist that I am allergic to nuts and legumes, which means I have to depend on animal protein. I still use the soy tempeh serum, but I don't eat soy tempeh anymore. Use common sense and refer to a nutritionist for more in- depth guidance.

This book has one serious juice recipe, but you can create so many wonderful juices of your own. Juicing is incredibly supportive of your immune system. Green juice, especially, reduces inflammation. It's worth it to get your own juicer instead of buying juice at the store. Naturally, you want to choose the freshest, cleanest organic ingredients you can find. Fresh food is still alive when you bring it home. No food in cans if you can possibly help it! Also, throw out anything that has been sitting in your refrigerator too long and looks faded, slimy, or wilted. Do not eat anything that you dropped on the floor! If you are really serious about preventing cancer, being conscientious counts. Avoiding those specks of dirt or decay means avoiding inflammation or other infections that your immune system does not need to deal with.

You may be aware that cold press and masticating juicers leave more of the enzymes intact because they cause less friction while juicing. The difference is definitely noticeable, so do what you can to find a good juicer. If you want to save money, buy a solid Omega or other well built juicer second hand - getting a cheap juicer new will only make you sad if it falls apart later!

The same can be said for your yogurt maker or Instant Pot. These tend to be less expensive than juicers. Do your research and get a quality yogurt maker, it doesn't have to be pricey but you will thank yourself later for investing the time.

Soy Tempeh Serum

Tempeh is made from soybeans fermented with fungi, either Rhizopus oryzae or Rhizopus oligosporus, of which R. oligosporus produces the most antioxidant and anti carcinogenic compounds.

The easiest way to get a concentrated dose of cancer-killing oligosporus compounds is to make Soy Tempeh Serum in your refrigerator. This yields a translucent liquid similar to the "water" in a yogurt container, and a clumpy, beige mass of solids at the bottom.

Try to find a brand of organic soy milk that has the least amount of additives possible, or, make your own soy milk!

Ingredients:

1/2 gallon container of organic, unsweetened unflavored soy milk 1 packet Tempeh starter (R. oligosporus)

Instructions:

Add the packet of tempeh starter to an airtight container of soy milk, such as a Mason jar. If you're using a container you bought from the store, it's very easy to keep it hygienic and culture only the oligosporus by opening the safety seal, putting in the tempeh starter, and closing the container lid tightly right away. Remember, it is always easier to practice good fermentation hygiene and get a clean culture using the store bought container of soy milk. Use meticulous sanitary practices, and if you aren't sure how, take a course in fermentation and/or canning to be safe. Shake the starter together with the soy milk. Leave in the refrigerator. After a few days, you can start pouring small amounts of serum to drink (1/4 cup or less). The serum will strengthen with time and keep indefinitely.

Quick Endocrine Balance Elixir

This Elixir is to elicit a quick response from your immune system to inflammation, pain, and discomfort that could eventually lead to cancer or be related to cancer cells. According to research, our bodies do have a certain number of cancer cells that occur naturally every day, and our immune system is central to killing those cells so the cancer can't reproduce. The Soy Tempeh Serum is "cytotoxic" to cancer cells, meaning that it kills them. This serum is fast acting and I have often used it when waking up in the middle of the night with painful inflammation or shooting pains, and gone back to get a good night's sleep afterwards.

Remember to drink some filtered water as a chaser, because it tastes HORRIBLE. It really does taste sour and kind of funky because of the kelp powder, but once it's in your tummy, it's going to make you FEEL great!

Ingredients:

1/4 cup soy tempeh serum
1 teaspoon kelp powder (Ascophylum nodosum) 1 teaspoon charcoal powder
1/4 teaspoon ashwaghanda powder
1/4 teaspoon powdered vitamin C
Instructions:
Measure all the ingredients into a glass. Add some water (I like to add warm water) and

stir. Drink it fast! Then drink some water and have a bite of something or some tea to get rid of the taste.

Tempeh Fermented Fruit

R. oligosporus can be used to ferment fruit as well, and fruit fermented with this fungus is loaded with compounds that kill cancer cells. However, fermenting fruit with oligosporus is time consuming and tricky to keep clean. If you decide to take the plunge and ferment fruit with oligosporus, the result is a jelly-like substance loaded with nutritious pectin that is super healthy for your digestion.

Ingredients:

8 oz of your choice from the following fruits:

Stone fruit (cherries, nectarines, peaches, apricots) Apple

Pear

Cranberries

Raspberries

Blueberries

Strawberries

Grapes

1/2 packet of tempeh starter dissolved in 1/4 cup water OR

1/4 cup of soy tempeh serum

Instructions:

Inoculate the whole fruit with the tempeh culture in a clean bowl by pouring in the dissolved starter/ serum and stirring gently to make sure the fruit is covered with the culture.

Put the fruit in a heat-safe bowl and incubate in a yogurt maker for at least 24 hours. You can also use an Instant Pot on the yogurt setting.
Remove when it starts to "gel" and takes on a translucent appearance. Enjoy! This is a very unique food for sure.

Homemade Soy Tempeh

Homemade tempeh is far cheaper than the store bought version. You can also switch up the ingredients and grow tempeh culture on brown or black rice!

"Hempeh", made with hemp seeds is another option, which does tend to be more expensive to make, with a mushier texture and more unconventional taste, but full of Omega-3 fatty acids and an acceptable substitute for those with soy allergies.

Ingredients:

4 cups dried organic soybeans

1 packet tempeh starter

1 1/2 quarts water

2 tablespoons organic rice vinegar 4 banana leaves, defrosted

OR

2 plastic ziplock bags

Instructions:

Boil the soybeans in the water until they are cooked. Just like pasta, you want to get just past the al dente stage and then drain the beans and rinse them.

Do your best to scoop out the bean hulls that come off during cooking. You can scoop them out with a ladle or sieve during cooking and using your clean hands after draining. This makes quite a bit of waste! It's far better to compost the hulls than it is to burden your garbage disposal with the fibrous hulls.

While the beans are still warm, pour in the rice vinegar and the tempeh starter. Stir well to make sure all of the soybeans are covered with the starter.

Then, pack the mixture into the banana leaves and wrap with a rubber band, or pack into the ziplock bags. Place the packed tempeh into your yogurt maker or Instant Pot and incubate on the yogurt setting for 24-48 hours. You can check on it every 12 hours or so, to see the white rhizomes of the fungus growing between the beans. Also, make sure there is a small amount of water in the bottom of the machine at all times, or the carbohydrates from the soy will burn! Turn the packets so they incubate evenly. Remove when the fungus has covered all the beans.

Ajo Sacha Tea

Ajo sacha is an Amazonian wonder herb. I first drank fresh ajo sacha in 2017 while visiting Peruvian Shipiba shaman Maestra Matilda in Nauta. The situation there is very rugged, with limited water for drinking/cleaning, and composting toilets. If that is too extreme for you, you can just order it on Etsy, there are quite a few sellers offering quality ajo sacha.

Ajo sacha is traditionally taken during a "dieta", or vegan/vegetarian fasting period (vegan is better for the cleanse if you can manage). 24 hours of dieta before taking a one-time dose of ajo sacha is enough. If you have a serious situation and need a deep cleanse, practice the dieta for one or two days before starting your course of ajo sacha and continue the dieta for as long as you are taking ajo sacha, up to two weeks.

You can NOT take ajo sacha every day indefinitely. Your body will be too drained. After a two week dieta, rest for at least one month before starting again.

No sex or alcohol are allowed during the dieta, as the chemicals involved reduce the efficacy of the herb. Ajo sacha will also make you sleepy and need to pee, so make sure you have time to rest. For example, take it after a light vegan lunch and make sure there is a clean bathroom nearby and that you have the afternoon free to nap. This recipe is meant to be taken once a day.

Ingredients:

4 tablespoons ajo sacha powder 1 quart of filtered water

Instructions:

Boil the powder in the filtered water for 20 minutes. Allow it to cool, but drink the entire quart at one sitting while it is still warm.

Anti-inflammation Breakfast Bowl

This is a breakfast açaí bowl that leaves out the granola, which can have refined sugars in it and other ingredients that cause inflammation. To compensate, it has extra superfood goodies and ingredients that are packed with antioxidants!

Ingredients:

1/4 cup pomegranate seeds

1/2 cup blueberry

1 açaí packet

2 tablespoons organic hemp seed 2 tablespoons raw cacao powder

OR

1/4 cup raw cacao nibs

1/4 teaspoon ashwaghanda 1/4 teaspoon turmeric

Instructions:

Combine all ingredients in a bowl. Enjoy with a warm tea or warm water to stimulate digestion and nutrient absorption.

Anti-inflammation Super Juice

The crowning achievement of this juice is the aloe vera cubes, which make the juice fun to drink, and at the same time provide deeply soothing glycoproteins, polyphenols, beta-carotene, huge amounts of vitamin C, magnesium, vitamin E, B12 and folic acid. Aloe vera has been linked to reduced risk of cancer, reduced inflammation, and reduced risk of diabetes, as well as increased hair growth!

So you know what to do...

Ingredients:

1 aloe vera leaf

1 bunch cilantro

1 cucumber

1 ounce fresh turmeric 1 ounce fresh ginger 1 lime

1 bunch spinach

1 apple

1/2 ounce wheatgrass

Instructions:

Cut the aloe vera leaf into two or three segments so that you don't have to cut the entire length of the leaf at once. Carefully slice the skin off of the gel. The skin is bitter, so just be aware that it will make your drink taste differently if you leave it in.

Next, cut the gel into small cubes and save them in a covered bowl. You can put them in the refrigerator to keep them cool if you like.

Take all the remaining ingredients and run them through your juicer. Then, add the aloe vera chunks. You can keep this in the refrigerator and drink whenever you need that glorious nutrient boost!

Inflammation Soothing Tea

A simple, non-caffeinated herbal tea that balances and reinvigorates. Ashwaghanda is an endocrine regulator that supports healthy hormone balance, while ginger, cardamom, and turmeric reduce inflammation, improve blood circulation, cleanse the liver, and support healthy digestion. Soursop leaf is known to contain compounds that help the body destroy cancer cells.

Ingredients:

1/4 teaspoon ashwaghanda powder 1/4 teaspoon cardamom powder 1/4 teaspoon turmeric powder

1 small piece of fresh ginger

2 soursop leaf pieces

Instructions:

Cut up the fresh ginger or use a vegetable peeler to shave it into small pieces. Put it in a cup with the soursop leaves. Add a little bit of water to prevent the powders from sticking to the bottom of your cup, then add the powders. Fill up with freshly boiled, filtered water. If you like, you may add honey and your favorite milk.

Liver Cleansing Tea

Cleansing the liver is very important because the liver eliminates toxins from our blood, often storing them to prevent them from circulating in our bodies. This tea helps flush those stored toxins from the liver.

Be aware that if you have never done a liver cleanse before, this tea may slow you way down when you first start drinking it. You may experience fatigue, diarrhea, and moodiness similar to PMS. Be sure to make enough time in your schedule to accommodate your need to rest and recover.

There are liver cleanses that you can buy at your local health food store that involve a specific diet plan and many more ingredients. I highly recommend those if you have the time (two weeks is the one I did) and can stick to the instructions about diet and when to take the tinctures and capsules. You will have so much more energy than you had before, you would be surprised!

Ingredients:

1 tablespoon milk thistle powder 1 tablespoon yarrow

1 tablespoon Angelica

Instructions:

Steep the herbs in hot water for five minutes. Let cool, then drink.

Toasted Tempeh Salad

This salad combines warm tempeh with cool fresh lettuce for a satisfying high-protein lunch or dinner.

Ingredients:

4 ounces of tempeh

4 or 5 large leaves of lettuce

2 carrots

1 piece of ginger

1 toe of garlic

1 shallot

1 tablespoon of coconut aminos 1 tablespoon rice vinegar

Instructions:

Cut the lettuce into bite size pieces and put in a bowl. Grate the carrots and ginger. Thin-slice the garlic and shallot. In a small bowl, combine the coconut aminos, vinegar, garlic and shallot. Gently toast the tempeh in a ceramic non-stick pan or air fryer until it is golden brown.

Combine all the ingredients in the bowl and enjoy!

Coconut Chicken With Vegetables

Coconut is one of nature's miracle foods. It is anti-inflammatory and a non-dairy source of healthy fats for those of us who react to lactose. It is a clean, green fuel for your cells, and it's also delicious!

Ingredients:

8 oz chicken breast

1 tablespoon coconut oil

1 cup of coconut milk or cream

2 sprigs of cilantro

1 large carrot

1 red pepper

2 large leaves of Swiss chard

1 piece of fresh ginger or galangal 2 kaffir

lime leaves (optional)

1 star anise pod

1/2 stalk of lemongrass

1/2 teaspoon of turmeric powder 1/4

teaspoon of salt

Instructions:

Chop the vegetables into bite size pieces, chop the chicken breast into bite size pieces and set aside.

Grate the ginger, then combine it in a sauce pan with the seasonings and coconut oil. Warm the seasonings in the oil.

Add the chicken and stir fry it in the coconut oil. When the chicken is cooked on the outside but pink on the inside, add the remaining ingredients, including the coconut milk and reduce the heat to a simmer. When the chicken is cooked all the way through, remove from heat. Serve with brown rice.

Bitter Melon Tofu with Purple Okinawan Sweet Potato

This recipe pays homage to the Okinawans, who famously live past 100 years old and remain free of chronic diseases like diabetes and cancer for their whole lives!

I've used tofu here, but the Okinawans traditionally eat freshly caught fish. It's up to you what protein you decide to use.

Bitter melon is one of those surprising foods that you never thought you would enjoy until you try cooking it at home. So many bitter melon dishes in restaurants are served with ajinomoto or other sauce thickeners that detract from the health benefits.

I went out of my way to find the seeds of the traditional Jyunpaku Okinawan bitter melon variety, which is supposed to be the tastiest, most savory bitter melon that can be eaten without cooking! Most bitter melon varieties that you find at the Asian grocery store have to be soaked in water to remove the bitterness, but not these tiny gourds, which have a translucent, lumpy white outer rind. If you like growing plants, you might try this one out.

Biting into one of these bitter melons is sort of like eating a pickle that is bitter instead of sour. It's a mildly enjoyable shock to the taste buds. But afterwards, when it hits the stomach, you experience a tiny but very distinct little rush. It's like an inspiration to sit up straight and take a deeper breath. I love it. I hope you enjoy it, too.

Ingredients:

1 bitter melon gourd

1/2 pound of silken tofu

1 tablespoon coconut oil

1 piece of fresh ginger

1 green onion

1 teaspoon Chinese five spice powder 1 tablespoon soy sauce.

1 purple okinawan sweet potato

Instructions:

Put the sweet potato in a steamer basket, double boiler or Instant Pot to steam.

Cut the tofu and the bitter melon into bite size pieces. Put the bitter melon into cold water if you want to reduce the bitterness. Dice the green onion. Then, heat the coconut oil in a nonstick pan until it sizzles. Add the tofu, the five spice and soy sauce, then turn the heat down to a simmer. When the tofu browns, turn it over. Then add the bitter melon and green onion. Stir fry this until the other side of the tofu browns.

Serve with the steamed sweet potato.

Anti-inflammation Poultice

Some of us get symptoms of inflammation or cancer on the outside. In my case, angry red blisters bubbled up through my skin and burned through the back of my neck. When this happens, our bodies are detoxifying by pushing toxins out through the skin.

This poultice is designed to chelate the toxins (with charcoal and magnesium) and help soothe and heal the skin (sea moss). You can also take this internally if you feel that your digestive tract is sore and inflamed from toxins.

Ingredients:

1/2 cup of Irish moss (sea moss)

1 pint of filtered water

1/2 cup of charcoal powder

4 tablespoons of magnesium powder

Instructions:

Soak the Irish moss in the water until it absorbs, usually overnight. The result is a gel interspersed with the stringy algae. Use a strainer to separate the gel from the algae, which you can throw away. Stir the charcoal powder and magnesium powder into the gel, and smear the mixture on the sore places. Leave it there until the skin cools down and starts to scab or close up. Then wipe with a damp cloth.

Stay hydrated and get lots of rest!

Blessings,

Malian

Made in the USA
Las Vegas, NV
05 February 2024

85333385R10036